MY LITTLE PINK NOTEBOOK

MY LITTLE PINK NOTEBOOK

How To Be Your Own Best Advocate Fighting Cancer & Other Monsters

Judi Klosek-Péladeau, JD

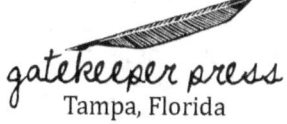
Tampa, Florida

The content associated with this book is the sole work and responsibility of the author. Gatekeeper Press had no involvement in the generation of this content.

MY LITTLE PINK NOTEBOOK: How To Be Your Own Best Advocate Fighting Cancer & Other Monsters

Published by Gatekeeper Press
7853 Gunn Hwy., Suite 209
Tampa, FL 33626
www.GatekeeperPress.com

Copyright © 2023 by Judi Klosek-Péladeau, JD
All rights reserved. Neither this book, nor any parts within it may be sold or reproduced in any form or by any electronic or mechanical means, including information storage and retrieval systems, without permission in writing from the author. The only exception is by a reviewer, who may quote short excerpts in a review.

The cover design and editorial work for this book are entirely the product of the author. Gatekeeper Press did not participate in and is not responsible for any aspect of these elements.

ISBN (paperback): 9781662944161

Contents

DEDICATION   1

1
THE BEGINNING & NOT THE END   3

2
DETOURS, SIDE TRIPS & MONSTERS   15

3
MISDIAGNOSIS   29

4
BIOPSY, HAZMAT SUIT & ONE CARING DOCTOR   39

5
SIDE EFFECTS, BIG PHARMA & SUPERCILIOUS DOCTORS   49

6
HUMORLESS PRACTITIONERS & LAUGHTER THERAPY   65

7
TRUE LOVE & FURRY FRIENDS   75

8
PRAY, PRAY & PRAY MORE   85

AFTERWORD   95
NOTES   97

DEDICATION

This book is dedicated to my dearest Mom, Dad and Sister, along with the thousands of other cancer warriors who get up each morning with pain, uncertainty, and the daunting reality of facing their own mortality.

1

THE BEGINNING & NOT THE END

"Keep your face to the sunshine and you cannot see the shadows. It's what sunflowers do."

—Helen Keller

This is my story—upfront, candid and very personal.

It is a love story of sorts with a very big twist. "My Little Pink Notebook" is definitely not about cancer, the disease, itself, or any of the associated scientific or medical jargon, but about the undefeated human spirit that refuses to give up in the face of adversity.

As a relentless researcher, I perused hundreds of books on the topic of cancer and found many of them dealt with very technical and scientific aspects of the disease. While there is a definite need for these books, I didn't find much encouragement, enlightenment, or helpful real-life insights on how to navigate through the exasperating healthcare institutions and frightening cancer roller coaster ride.

This is the book I wanted to read during my fight against breast cancer, but couldn't find it in any bookstore, library, or e-book. So I wrote it!

To survive a trauma like cancer, you really have to be able to tell a story about it. Everyone's journey is unique and packed with incredible emotional turmoil, both physical and mental highs and lows, and as all the warriors I met along the way confided in me, filled with a lot of faith, hope, love and prayer. What I definitely know leads to ultimate victory is a positive mindset, accompanied by undying faith, love, joy and laughter, wherever and whenever you can grab it.

Putting both the magnitude of cancer and its impact on human beings in perspective, consider that worldwide each year around 18.1 million individuals will receive a cancer diagnosis, 10 million will die from the disease, and 7.4 million will be misdiagnosed.

Reportedly, five percent of cancers are caused by genetic mutations; sixty-six percent by random errors that occur during the ongoing natural process of cellular division; a large percentage develops due to unknown causes.

Patients often beat themselves up thinking it's something they did wrong, but cancer is its own Rubik's Cube—complex and difficult to solve. It is unpredictable, has a will of its own, and is a fierce enemy with the power to take over the 30 trillion plus cells in your body. Deceptively, it may go into hiding for years and come back with vengeance when you least expect it.

Some patients may be fortunate to get an accurate early diagnosis; others may not; many receive the correct diagnosis, too late, after the cancer has spread to other body parts, resulting in long-term harm, or death.

It is no wonder that cancer has been labelled, "Emperor of all maladies." While I remain hopeful that someday there will be a total cure, in the current state of medical science, this disease continues to be one of life's most threatening monsters.

While these statistics sound grim, the very positive message throughout my notebook is that you never have to allow the disease to invade your spirit or soul. You're in control of that domain!

Keep in mind cancer stats are just numbers, and don't even begin to tell the true story. Behind the data are real humans, maybe your family members, your friends, or yourself. Among these statistics were my own Mom, Dad and Sister. My Dad's cancer was misdiagnosed; Mom's was caught after it was inoperable. Fortunately, my Sister beat the odds.

These are my real heroes. They were the compelling impetus to write and to share my notebook, chronicling my own ongoing cancer journey, experiences, insights, family stories, and hard-learned lessons, as I found myself smack in the middle of one of the most serious shortcomings of the healthcare system—misdiagnosis.

During my family's battle with the "big C," they taught me the importance of love, internal strength, staying in control, and keeping focused on life's purpose, while never losing a sense of joy and good humor.

I clearly remember in one of the many candid talks I had with my Dad, a former Chief in the New York City Fire Department, when I bluntly asked him while he was on his deathbed, "What does it feel like to die?" Without skipping a beat, in his very weak, raspy, hardly audible voice, he replied, "Have you ever been to Cleveland in the scorching heat of summer?" I laughed heartily, along with the family members around his bedside. Dad never allowed his cancer to diminish his incredible humor, wit, or corny jokes. Like a spoonful of sugar, he always helped any bitter medicine, life struggle, or sad news go down a little easier.

Not to be outwitted by my Dad, Mom had an equally wry sense of Brooklyn, New York humor. One day while visiting her at the nursing home, she told me jokingly, "The difference between the terrifying Coney Island cyclone ride and cancer is that the roller coaster fright only lasts ten minutes." *Bada-Bing Bada-Boom!*

I am unapologetic for calling out some physicians, practitioners, and institutions for their uncaring attitudes, poor communications and unacceptable health management practices that place priority on time management and profit, over patient-focused medical practices.

After all is said and done, is it not every doctor's duty under the Hippocratic Oath to put patients' health and healing first, and do everything medically possible to make their patients healthy?

I celebrate many of the remarkable medical advances, and acknowledge the scientific breakthroughs continually occurring in cancer research. I loudly applaud those doctors who practice medicine with genuine care, thoroughness, and professionalism, focused on making patients better, not just prescribing drugs. But, In addition to the unacceptable encounters I experienced with some medical establishments, I sadly remember specific conversations with a few doctors who told me their patient caseload prevented them from being as thorough as needed. One doctor from a private healthcare hospital confided that his annual bonus was partially based on the number of diagnostic tests and costs he kept down.

Some of these startling revelations were confirmed in a 2022 Kaiser Union survey that indicated the top reasons given by physicians for leaving their practices were the unsustainable workloads and administrative directives that interfered with their ability to deliver the quality standard of care needed for every patient.

Even the American Medical Association's, "Moving Medicine" podcast, a strong voice in healthcare, forecasts one out of five doctors will leave the profession over the next five years due to burnout and institutional regulations which often interfere with a doctor's ability to provide quality care. Not only is the healthcare system, itself, in peril, but all patients face worrisome and serious consequences from these failing systems.

In stark contrast, can you imagine the absolutely positive impact on patients if medical institutions rewarded doctors for putting patients first, for keeping patients healthy, for making sure all treating physicians have reasonable workloads, and, additionally, providing all the critical state-of-art tools, incentives and support necessary?

Based on my medical odyssey and real-life experiences, where I sometimes faced uncaring practitioners, along with disjointed coordination with other necessary professional services, I believe there is a crucial need for a truly seamless, multi-disciplinarian approach to patient care. While much of the healthcare institutional and public relations literature proclaim they are "integrated, multi-disciplinary, and the patient is at the center of their healthcare" few live up to this promise. Concurrently, there is an urgent need for a total paradigm shift, concentrated on treating patients as whole persons—body, mind and spirit.

On the horizon, as more and more scientific breakthroughs and technologies put increasing focus on robotic procedures and artificial intelligence (AI), my plea is that the human programmers and engineers behind these cutting-edge technologies make absolutely certain humanistic treatment of patients is primary. As the expression goes, once the genie is out of the bottle, it isn't going to be easy to get it back in and control its actions.

Patients must rally now for making more humanistic patient treatment a top priority.

HAL 9000, the artificial intelligence, talking, controlling character, and main antagonist many of us met decades ago in Stanley Kubrick's, "2001: Space Odyssey" must be kept in check since over the years, he has grown extremely powerful, more intelligent, and formidable.

Artificial Intelligence is by no means inherently bad, and offers great promise for diagnostic use and application in many areas of medicine. In fact, a recent medical study from Sweden showed that AI was twenty percent more effective than doctors in the early detection of breast cancer. Nevertheless, patients must strongly advocate for putting human control over machines, and become actively involved in the current social debate, making sure robots are used only as tools and medical assistants to doctors. We must have ethical humans, not machines, as leaders who possess the moral clarity to know the difference between right and wrong, making critical decisions impacting the human race.

Hard-Learned Lesson:

Cancer is a tough teacher! Prepare yourself to be an even tougher and relentless self-advocate.

2

DETOURS, SIDE TRIPS & MONSTERS

> *"It is never your enemies that defeat you, but your own fear of the bullies and monsters in your life that will take you down."*
>
> —Dad

Many magnificent golden and purple moons ago in Hawaii, when my husband, Charles, and I traveled on vacation to the Big Island, we had no idea we were embarking on the most exciting and challenging adventures of our lifetime. The experience created a lasting memory of emotions—many positively great, some bad, and a few ugly. As the great philosopher Aristotle taught, everything happens for a reason, and it wasn't until decades later that this life event became extremely relevant to my struggle with cancer. It not only highlighted, but underscored the fact that cancer is only one single chapter in your life, among a multitude of happy, colorful, fun and rich ones.

We were in desperate need of R&R. I just passed the California State and Hawaii State Bar exams after finishing a grueling 18 month accelerated law school degree at Southwestern University School of Law. Charles gave up his very demanding and successful string of Jiu-jitsu schools back in Ontario, Canada, where he had won the Canadian National Championship, earning him a strong student following, and an enviable reputation as a Nidan Black Belt.

Without any itinerary or time schedule, not even an AAA road map, we enthusiastically packed our bags to replenish our souls and escape the 24-hour frenzy of the Los Angeles freeways and lifestyle. Before leaving for the islands, I even dutifully had my annual mammogram. Everything seemed perfect; there was no trace of breast cancer, an ongoing concern based on recurring cysts. What an enormous relief!

When we finally got to the Big Island, we felt we had reached the Garden of Eden. The Mamalahoa Scenic Highway, the main road, is so diverse in its landscape with each part of the three hundred mile stretch filled with overgrown eucalyptus and tropical trees, forming an enchanting lush green canopy.

It was an exquisite getaway for two Californian burned-out souls. Instantly, we became totally absorbed in the unique flora and fauna and entered into a Zen-like trance, becoming one with the tropical surroundings. When we finally reached the northern coast of the island, an overwhelming mysterious force overtook us, as if we drank from one of the "Alice in Wonderland" magical potions.

After traveling several hours, stopping only once to taste the local favorite cuisine of loco mocos, and sumptuous warm malasadas, our uncontrollable curiosity compelled us to turn into the first side road we crossed. It was a crooked and winding path that led us down a road definitely less traveled. Instant spontaneity was the only explanation for this detour. It wasn't until years later, like so many things that happen to us, that we realized it was one of the most significant side trips of our lifetime. And, little did I know, or even suspect, it would prepare me for my battle later in life with one of life's biggest detours.

The Hamakua coastline is a rich lush tropical rainforest with stunning greenery and melodious birds chirping in harmony in what seem like orchestrated sound effects with the nearby waterfalls spilling into the landscape. The air was filled with deliciously sweet and intoxicating flowers producing the most magnificent smells. We were under a tropical spell!

Continuing to travel at a snail's pace down the side roads, we made another screeching halt when we saw an old abandoned café and gas station, frozen in time. We immediately pulled over, got out of the car, brushed aside the thick dust and cobwebs covering the cracked window and peeked inside the old structure, hugging the side of the rough road. Our imaginations went wild. Much to our wondrous eyes, we saw a magnificent soda fountain, something right out of 1950s. We thought it must have been where the town's people gathered decades ago over a strawberry ice cream, or chocolate malt and juicy burger. At least in our imagination, it had to be the past social media center of the town, pre-dating anything even closely resembling today's chic Starbucks cafés. We could almost hear the local town gossip and smell the beef, procured from the local cattle ranches, cooking on the old rusty grill. With our noses still glued to the window, we saw a long faded red Formica countertop, a rusty old ice cream freezer and malt mixer. We strained our necks even further to see into a connecting doorway, where we saw what appeared to be a corroded old stove. Indeed, it was a trip back to the 50s, and a soon-to-be-life-changing dramatic experience.

Our still out-of-control curiosity beckoned us about a hundred yards further down the road where we spotted an old house that looked occupied. We approached the house, knocked on the door, and a weathered old man came to the front door. I blurted out, "Do you know anything about that old café? Looking extremely puzzled and suspicious, the man reluctantly nodded and said that he was the owner of the property. In a very unfriendly voice he asked, "What do you want?" I said, "Could you show us the place?" He hesitated for a few minutes, turned back into the house, and much to our surprise, came back with a key, told us to go inside the café and be sure to knock on his door when we were finished looking.

After checking every square inch of the dilapidated café, we went back to the owner's house and asked if he would consider renting us the café. More confused-looking than before, he asked us why we wanted it and what we would do with it. After an unbelievably short period of time by any measure for negotiating a business deal, we ended up signing a simple handwritten contract for what was to become our dream café. It was by far the quickest, craziest and most spontaneous decision of our marriage, but it felt very right.

After signing the agreement, we decided to end our Hamakua road travels on the spot and drove about 20 miles back to the main town of Hilo; rented a studio in a nearby local hotel; extended our sketchy timeline; put a major restoration plan in place. After severing ties in California, we went to work turning our exciting discovery into a wonderful re-creation of an old 1950s café. Turquoise painted walls, country curtains, and checkered tablecloths, with tons of memorabilia from the past, turned it into a fantasy café. The only modern touch was a great Bose sound system that continuously played the smooth swing sounds of Billie Holiday, Louis Armstrong and all the old songs of the 50s from "I Only Have Eyes for You" to "At the Hop" and "Don't Be Cruel," which we often danced to the music, along with folks who visited the café. The pièce de résistance, the finishing touch, was a huge colorful hand-made sign painted by a local artist, depicting a happy caricature of a dancing Hawaiian couple.

We hung it outside the café next to a flashing neon sign that read: "Open." It was our "Field of Dreams." We built it and they definitely came. Over the weeks ahead, we attracted a multitude of local residents and tourists. We called our re-creation, The Local Café of Laupahoehoe, after the name of the town which had a population of only 450 people, climbing to over 1000 residents today.

While Charles did all the heavy work reconstructing the place, I went to work preparing news releases, articles and announcements in all the newspapers from Honolulu to San Francisco, Los Angeles, New York and points beyond. Literally, we put the café on the map. Eventually, we appeared in Frommer's travel books, and other top tourist guidebooks on Hawaii, along with articles appearing in major newspaper travel sections. It was not only the uniqueness of the

Local Café of Laupahoehoe, the unexpected surprise of a lively and colorful replica of a 50s café, tucked away on the Hamakua coast where there was little to do other than gaze at the dramatic scenery, but the appetites of hungry travelers who came for our famous Colossal Burgers, both fresh beef and veggie. We were told by our local patrons that our food *broke da mouth*, a popular colloquial expression, meaning yummy. We even created a mini replica museum, depicting the history of the old plantation days the coastal area was known for in the 40s and 50s.

As fate would have it, the Local Café of Laupahoehoe turned out to be a smashing successful tourist destination, bringing people from all over the island, the mainland and even overseas. But, it was a bittersweet success. Our notoriety and popularity created envy and jealousy among some of the local residents who started *talking stink*, trashing our business sign, ransacking parts of our business property, and trying to attack us personally in an attempt to literally drive us off the road while we drove on the highway. This simply occurred because we were *haoles*—a disparaging term rooted in a deep-seated prejudice against people not born, or raised in Hawaii. When we turned to the local police for help, they refused to assist because of their incestuous ties to the community. By all accounts told to us by our more supportive and friendly local patrons, a cadre of vicious locals, very jealous of our success and hell-bent on running us out of town, led the attacks. The enemy had arrived in the form of small town treacherous bullies who attacked when we weren't looking, mostly at night.

The stress started taking its toll. I started having horrendous nightmares. After months of these bully monsters attacking Charles and me, continually through the middle of my deep sleep, I knew I had to come up with an immediate solution. I decided to create a counter-monster, actually a super-hero, bigger, more powerful, and capable of stopping the surreptitious nightly assaults. So one night when the bad dream recurred, I would be prepared this time with my counter offensive strategy in place. I was getting ready to deploy my own Goliath.

As I vividly recall, my monster was a much larger and aggressive adaptation of the giant "Michelin Man," one of the oldest commercial tire trademarks which depicted a giant stack of white super puffy tires. During that time, the tire commercial appeared everywhere on TV and, obviously, imprinted a strong and lasting impression on me. My dream battle with the enemy ensued and acted as my personal super-hero, a version of the "Michelin Man," who fiercely confronted, ferociously attacked, and defeated the enemy monster, right in the middle of my sleep.

Dream researchers and psychologists would probably claim that my dream was a powerful unconscious solution to a major unresolved real-life threat. It helped me navigate the situation away from the actual dangerous situation, and allowed me safely to come up with a creatively effective strategy to end, once and for all, the actual ugly situation.

It worked! I never had that bad dream again. While the real local villains continued their criminal attacks, we became more psychologically and physically prepared to expose their tactics with one of modern days most powerful weapons—a video and sound camcorder which caught them cold-handed. A big victory! This time I went over the heads of the local colluding police right to the Chief of Police in Hilo with the incriminating evidence in hand. The video clearly captured the locals' unlawful acts and forced the Chief to stop the assaults. Double victory!

To this day, whenever I sense I am being bullied, or harassed, I send in my hero monster to defeat the pain, the stress, even the unwelcomed side effects caused by the "big C" monster. My strategy, which was originally embedded in a deep dream state, continues to work as a powerful real-life psychological tool to help defeat negative thoughts, experiences, and assuage the fear of unexpected attacks.

I'm sure a dream interpreter would further acknowledge that this mental device works because it puts me in control, switches my role from victim to victor, and strengthens my resolve to stay strong and win.

Hard-Learned Lesson:

You always have two choices: give up and be defeated, or fight cancer, along with all the other big ugly monsters you run into in your life. Those beasts can never destroy your soul or spirit, unless you let them. My dream adaptation of the "Michelin Man" became a metaphor for the courage to stand up to all the ruffians in life, in all their many forms and disguises. Create your own!

A strong mental resolve and unbeatable determination to overcome the bad stuff in your life will lead you to eventual victory, no matter what the outcome. Both your unconscious and subconscious mindset matters. So do pay close attention to your dreams!

3

MISDIAGNOSIS

"I am not afraid of the storms for I am learning how to navigate my ship."

—Louisa May Alcott

I was living the American dream back in California, flourishing in my career and personal life, trying to embrace all that was positive and joyful. Unannounced, without warning, cancer very sneakily, like a thief in the middle of the night, showed up. It tried to take me down and change my life's journey.

My uncontrollable pain was transforming me from a happy and balanced person into a pain-ridden and irrational one. I told my husband not to consider me a coward if I committed some dastardly act to end the pain. Sounding a lot like Lady Macbeth in Shakespeare's play, I repeatedly cried, "Out damn spot!" I pleaded with God for help to get rid of my insidious pain, relentlessly gnawing away at the intense spot in my right shoulder.

Four years earlier, I had no clue when my localized tumor was surgically removed from my right breast that it would resurface and travel the most expeditious route to my right shoulder. It seemed implausible, especially since all my doctors repeatedly told me during all my ongoing medical checkups that I was totally cancer-free, all margins were clear, no spread to lymph nodes.

I believed the doctors. I was home free; so I thought.

Pain can be a very powerful negative force on both the body and the mind. On the brink of my pain tolerance, I started thinking back over past decades, and thanked my lucky stars for the greatest, most devoted parents and the good nuns at St. Pancras Catholic School in Queens, New York, where I attended grammar school.

They taught me critical life lessons, values, virtues and the importance of staying strong when faced with any adversity. At my moment of extreme agony, this solid upbringing helped enormously, and prevented me from thinking of doing anything drastic to myself. Instead, it fortified me to keep fighting and moving forward for a positive and effective solution.

I don't remember many of my academic lessons in grade school, what day Paul Revere rode his horse through the American colonies, warning the settlers that the British were about to attack, or who everyone of the signers to the Declaration of Independence were, but I never forgot Sister Mary's dire warnings of the heinous consequences of any type of mortal sin, such as suicide. Those lessons were indelibly imprinted and drilled further into my developing childhood brain every Sunday during Mass conducted by Monsignor Pfeiffer of the parish church. While most of the nuns were truly loving and caring, in comparison, the Monsignor was harsh, uncaring and lived a privileged life. Even though he was ordained as an earthly representative of God, he took great pride in using cruel tactics to punish his young parishioners for the slightest offense. The most innocent crime, whispering in church, resulted in the offending child ordered by him to kneel in the church aisle for the entire hour-long Mass. His repeated refrain, "Depart from me you cursed into the flames of everlasting Hell," at the end of every sermon, was designed to remind church-goers that they were hopeless sinners, and served to drastically increase the impact of his terrorizing speeches. I could only imagine what punishment he would dole out if anyone dared to commit a really serious sin, and periodically pictured him in the afterlife, standing at the Pearly Gates with a stern face and arms tightly crossed, unmercifully delivering the everlasting and final punishment of Hell. It was a fierce image and powerful deterrent for anyone at any age!

Later in life when I became a lawyer, I couldn't help but speculate that the legal doctrine of proportionality— *the punishment must fit the crime—* was developed in response to this very mean Monsignor, whose reprisals were not only way out of whack and unsuitable for small offenses, but ungodly!

As my wise Dad told me, the Monsignor's personal life was far from holy, and in complete violation of his priesthood vows of poverty, chastity and obedience. This was a conclusion he must have easily drawn from seeing the pastor wearing fine clothing, driving around town in a big new black Cadillac, accompanied by a female companion. Dad always said, "What's important is to listen carefully and focus on the solid universal truths, principles and values you are being taught, and don't be negatively affected by a flawed priest's behavior, or by a misguided teacher delivering the words." He was right, as usual.

After fruitless doctor appointments and physical therapy sessions for over a year, by early 2020, I couldn't raise my right arm even the slightest, couldn't dress myself, couldn't sleep since the intense knife-like 24/7 stabbing pain was intolerable. On a scale of zero to ten, it broke the scale!

I went back to my primary care doctor at Kaiser Permanente and begged him to reassess the cause of my extreme pain. He continued to be dismissive and insisted it was *frozen shoulder*, a diagnosis he confirmed over and over again, and wrote a prescription for a stronger narcotic. Then, he said, "People at your age often get frozen shoulder." That did it! It was those words, "people at your age." It was ageism at its best. Again, he was ignoring my extreme pain, and chalking up my symptoms to age, without addressing the severity of my medical situation. I was tired of him gaslighting me, dismissing my complaints, and not seriously listening to me.

I was angry, frustrated, and very upset, but it was the exact big kick in the derrière I needed. I went into a strong self-advocacy mode, and I became determined to find a doctor who would get to the root of what was causing my pain, not just rely on drugs to ease the pain.

After doing research, I found a top-rated orthopedic surgeon outside of Kaiser, called his office for an appointment, and waited three long weeks to fit into his busy schedule. The MRI the doctor immediately ordered revealed a sizable lesion in my right shoulder. As he was examining the image of my shoulder, he declared without hesitation, "It looks like a cancerous tumor." I asked him, "How sure are you?" He said, "Pretty sure, but I can't confirm it until you get a biopsy, and I cannot even consider any further treatment until we know for sure if it is cancer."

This was the first time cancer was mentioned in connection with my right shoulder. The word reverberated like a disharmonious gong. Simultaneously, a shrill deafening sound went off in my head. I was in shock. The doctor repeated, "The only way to be sure it's cancer is to get your shoulder biopsied." He then asked, "Did you ever have breast cancer?" I was extremely puzzled that he seemed to be making a connection between my breast and shoulder.

I responded, "Yes, I did four years ago and had a complete right breast mastectomy and lymph nodes removed. The final diagnosis made by the surgeon was that I was free of cancer, the margins surrounding the excised tumor were clear, and nearby lymph nodes showed absolutely no signs of cancer." He said that may have been true four years ago, and insisted I contact the operating surgeon to make sure she urgently ordered a biopsy of my shoulder, and made my previous pathology report available for further study.

I was devastated. 7.4 million misdiagnoses happen each year. Now, pursuing my own treatment, I became another statistic, just one number among millions, running smack into the middle of one of the most severe systematic shortcomings of our healthcare system—misdiagnosis.

During my research, I found a study conducted by the Commonwealth Fund, a private global foundation seeking to promote high standards in healthcare, which reported Americans receive the worse health outcomes overall among the top 38 high-income nations of the world, and further it indicated that Americans' life expectancy is currently dropping. This ghastly reality is occurring despite the astronomical dollars, to the tune of 4.3 trillion dollars, spent each year on healthcare in the United States.

Something is amiss; something is very wrong. Patients must wake up, pay close attention to their medical treatment and healthcare institutions, and become very pro-active in managing their health. Certainly, never blindly trust the healthcare system.

Hard-Learned Lesson:

Every storm teaches us a powerful lesson. Take immediate action! Don't wait! Always get a second medical opinion as soon as possible if you have even the slightest inkling your doctor is not providing a thorough and accurate diagnosis. Don't stop pursuing the right solution until you get the correct diagnosis and treatment.

Just because someone has the designation of doctor before his or her name doesn't assure high-quality care, competency, or an accurate diagnosis. Take very good notes, keep records, and ask a lot of questions about the level and type of medical treatment you are receiving. In the long run, you are the best arbiter of your health and know best how your body is responding to treatment. You must become your own best advocate.

4

BIOPSY, HAZMAT SUIT & ONE CARING DOCTOR

"Every strike brings me closer to a home run"

—Babe Ruth

It was the beginning of the 2020 COVID pandemic. Healthcare systems were in disarray. The admitting nurse at Kaiser Hospital told me I was very lucky to get rushed into the system since the administrators were putting most procedures on hold unless they were life-or-death situations. "Lucky?" I replied. "I am here for a bone biopsy of my right shoulder for possible metastatic breast cancer since my family physician misdiagnosed my excruciating shoulder pain for over a year, and erroneously reassured me not to worry since it was simply frozen shoulder." No response from the nurse, but, nonetheless, I patiently waited for the doctor to do an X-ray-guided biopsy, while I was in a semi-sedated state, lying on a very chilly, hard, and narrow hospital gurney. I was number two patient in-waiting.

An hour later when it was my turn for the procedure, the doctor came by, introduced himself, and asked how I was doing. I said, "I feel like I am hanging off a cliff in suspense with no rescue team in sight. Doctor, do you think it is cancer?" He very nonchalantly replied, "Based on your X-rays and MRI, there is a strong possibility, but soon we will know for sure."

Three weeks later I was sitting in another sterile waiting room, euphemistically referred to by patients as "God's waiting room." This time I was sent to the Kaiser Cancer Treatment Center since the biopsy confirmed I had fourth stage metastatic breast cancer that traveled to my right shoulder.

The room was filled with a number of patients who looked very sick and worried. Forcing myself to be positive and hopeful in this bleak situation, I tried to convince myself that the other patients looked much worse than I did. Just then, the nurse came out, ushered me into a very small hermitically-sealed room with no windows, insisted I wear a double face mask, and explained that the doctor treating me would meet me through a computerized video camera due to the current COVID restrictions—an explanation I would hear repeatedly over the next year.

In reality, the doctor was in the room just next door to me, but because of these severe pandemic precautions, he was not allowed to meet with me face-to-face. When his image showed up on my computer monitor, he was introduced by an automated loud warning bell. I was directed by a voice recording to adjust my volume and video screen if the sound and picture weren't clear. Adding to the already tense situation, when the mystery doctor finally appeared on the screen, he was wearing what looked like a white Hazmat suit, covering him head to toe. His attire seemed extreme for the situation since we were in separate rooms. His voice was very muffled, probably because of the white protective armor totally covering his face.

The remoteness, coldness, lack of human contact, and sterility of the environment were unnerving. I didn't know if I was talking to a robot, a real doctor, or Doctor Strangelove.

As I adjusted the volume, the chill in my isolated room was somewhat ameliorated by his kind sounding voice and very apologetic words about the computer interface. After asking me a series of questions about my pain level and overall current health, I said, "Doctor, please cut to the chase and tell me what's in store for me; will I have to get radiation or chemotherapy; will the cancer rapidly move to other parts of my body; how much longer do I have to live? All I was told by previous doctors is that my previous right breast cancer moved to my right shoulder, even though I was repeatedly told for over four years that I was cancer-free."

At that moment, the doctor took off his multiple masks, stood up, and quite unexpectedly, said, "I'm coming in."

Was I ever surprised! I felt I was being rescued by Superman, or a messenger from God. He apparently decided to dispense with the extreme restrictions and meet with me in a more humanistic manner. When he entered my room, he cautiously sat well over six feet away from me and proceeded to ask a lot of personal questions which made me feel more like a human being he was concerned about, not just a cancer statistic. For the first time during the entire ordeal, I was being treated by a caring doctor who wanted to know more about me as a person, which should be standard protocol, but, unfortunately, is not. He told me the bad news that I would have to receive the highest dosage of targeted radiation medically allowable, with the initial goal of alleviating my ongoing agonizing shoulder pain.

After meticulously positioning me in a humongous futuristic-looking machine that would deliver the radiation through photon beams, and permanently tattooing the targeted right shoulder cancer spot, he explained that I would have to wait four weeks to see if the radiation treatment worked before any further treatments were ordered.

Despite this continued wait-and-see news, I was somewhat relieved that no chemotherapy was ordered, yet, and I was finally talking face-to-face with a real doctor. When we were finished conversing about next steps, I left the room feeling a bit more confident because of this doctor's personable approach, even though I still faced radiation and a lot of uncertainty as to what was next. With his caring manner, he sparked a strong positive response within me.

While I was driving home, I couldn't help but think of a wonderful show I saw years ago. The movie, "Patch

Adams," starring the late Robin Williams, put a very upbeat and positive twist on how medicine should be practiced. This true story was based on a remarkable doctor who had a dream to build a fully integrated holistic hospital which not only offered top quality medical care, but provided compassionate and joyful patient treatment.

The movie delivered a very strong message and an equally powerful punch in the gut to traditional medical establishments.

Paraphrasing Dr. Patch's impassioned and unforgettable monologue, he asked hospital administrators to change their way of thinking and revamp their existing paradigm of patient care which failed to put patients first, lacked humanistic care, good humor, and any trace of fun and love. He rightfully claimed that all these elements should be critical aspects of healing. And, in the very dramatic ending of his speech, he tearfully begged medical administrators and number crunchers, who run these institutions, to look at each and every patient as a whole person with emotions and feelings, and not only as a disease.

After my visit with one caring doctor, this poignant speech became more real than ever, and the truth of the message clearly cried out for the need for change in today's traditional medical practices.

Hard-Learned Lesson:

The clear lesson is to insist on being treated as a whole human being, not just as a disease. The bland and colorless medical environments, staffed too often by super-serious personnel, can be unhealthy and might even make you sicker!

Remember to bring a positive book with you, or a happy friend. Wear colorful clothing which will help lighten up your spirits and, most certainly, the dull and colorless waiting rooms.

5

SIDE EFFECTS, BIG PHARMA & SUPERCILIOUS DOCTORS

"Once you choose hope, anything is possible."

—Christopher Reeves/Superman

If you live on Planet Earth and watch TV, you can't help but be disturbed by the onslaught of commercials from Big Pharma on so-called wonder drugs, along with a multitude of other medical supplements and remedies, marketed and sold by them. No doubt, what concerns you most are not just the curative claims of the specific product advertised, but the long, scary litany of side effects associated with most drugs.

Try to recall any one drug you saw on TV and its sales pitch. You will probably become agitated thinking about the potential harmful impact it could have on your body. Obviously, prudence still dictates that you should always evaluate the benefits of any drug versus any negative effects which stand in the way of reaching a desired health outcome.

To make a fully informed decision, you need thorough information and truthful disclosures from the pharmaceutical companies.

It's very confusing and frustrating for most people to keep up with science, let alone the maze of constantly changing information coming from Big Pharma. Think about all the recent conflicting information surrounding the COVID vaccine, which sparked an epidemic of misinformation, based on unclear medical advice, uncertainty and, even, alleged conspiracy theories. Just recently a major news network reported a story that said among certain patients, heart attacks and deaths were directly associated with the vaccine.

You are definitely not being cynical or neurotic asking the tough questions to your doctor and demanding critical information from Big Pharma.

Over 4,500 FDA approved drugs are recalled each year in the United States, after being widely prescribed, ingested, injected, or implanted. These include a long-list of well-publicized drugs, from the disastrous Thalidomide, which caused serious birth defects, to Fen-phen and Vioxx, which resulted in heart problems and death. Recently the US Department of Justice exposed the extreme seriousness of the opioid crisis in America, and criminally charged Purdue Pharma and others for supplying opioids, without a legitimate medical purpose. Add to these incidences the ongoing controversy over the COVID vaccines, no wonder there is widespread public distrust of Big Pharma.

Twenty four hours after receiving the second dose of the Pfizer COVID vaccination, I had a mild heart attack and blood clot in my leg. Previously, I had absolutely no signs of heart disease, or clotting issues. Yet, doctors who treated me told me that they couldn't be sure those life-threatening side effects were caused by the vaccine. A year later, numerous medical reports indicated other patients had very similar dangerous side effects caused by the vaccine.

With all the ongoing controversy and politicization over the vaccines, it is understandable that many consumers are very reluctant to get the COVID booster shots being promoted by the drug companies.

Was Big Pharma covering up the side effects, while continuing to aggressively market and sell these drugs?

Using a simpler fictitious illustration, let's look at how a much less controversial drug for pain relief named "No Wonder" is marketed to the public. The actor representing the company begins by enthusiastically extolling the incredible, almost miraculous benefits, that can make you pain free in just days, or weeks, after years of experiencing agonizing pain. The announcer of this product, often a well-known actor, or TV personality, specifically chosen to try to generate automatic trust, explains how you'll be able to walk, hike, run, and move like you never did before. Then, the advertisement shows the spokesperson, after taking the pills, bouncing up from her favorite easy chair, without any signs of stiffness, or malady of any kind, running in the park, hiking in the wilderness, or dancing with her grandkids. Despite the credibility the actor is attempting to instantly create, you weren't born last night and know very well what appears too good to be true is probably not true. These sales pitches, both unrealistic and humorous, at best, can be very deceptive to the public.

Without debating the issue at length, I think you will agree that rarely are the promised results, as advertised, instantly achieved. The climax of the TV Ad always offers a big disclaimer, accompanied by a long list of side effects. All the information is read in record-speed, like an auctioneer selling cattle. The announcer cites the proverbial side effects list again which we've heard many times, including nausea, dizziness, blood clots, heart attacks, strokes, diarrhea, constipation, severe thirst, nightmares, sweats, high blood pressure, hallucinations, compulsive behaviors, or worse, could turn you into a sleep-walking zombie, or an alien with extra appendages.

You get the picture and heard it multiple times! After listening to these outrageous claims and hearing the terrifying report, no one would blame any reasonable person for skipping the drugs and living with the pain.

Remember, Big Pharma is comprised of for-profit companies and are constantly promoting their drugs to doctors who lean heavily on pharmaceutical solutions. The job of any publicly-traded company is to maximize the returns to their investors. Keeping it real, let's face it, the more diseases and viruses that invade our bodies, the more money these companies make. Accusing them of being greedy is like accusing zebras of having too many stripes. They are money-making businesses supposedly doing their job. We can't change that fact.

So what is our job? It is definitely the obligation of doctors and medical institutions, as well as our individual responsibility as patients, to insist that guardrails be put in place to ensure these companies, incorporated to serve our health needs, are fully transparent, honest, open, thorough, and disclose all harmful side effects, even those adverse effects which may cast serious public doubt on their use.

Along with your treating physician, you must be absolutely certain that the scientific research and clinical-base facts of all available drugs are accurate, complete and based on independent peer review, not just the information from the pharmaceutical manufacturing the drug, which can be absolutely skewed in their favor.

It is not my intention, or goal to denigrate the many incredible scientific and pharmaceutical advances that have been made in cancer treatments and other areas of medicine, which seem to work miracles, but to make sure you fully evaluate every drug prescribed and ingested in view of your overall health conditions, tolerances, and medical goals.

I am simply trying to shed light on the critical importance of honest communications with all your medical doctors, practitioners, and pharmacists before taking any prescribed drugs.

Based on my experience, these critical discussions around the drugs and treatments ordered, were often overlooked, downplayed, or omitted altogether.

As a patient, you always have choices and must demand full disclosures so that no drug can irreversibly harm you, or conflict with other prescriptions. If you are not able to make those decisions, make sure you have someone designated to help you.

So why are doctors too often unwilling to discuss the side effects? Are they just trying to be diplomatic and attempting to mitigate your fears so you don't run out of their office screaming in tears? Are they deliberately underestimating the potential problems that are associated with drugs? Or, are they just looking at you as a mere cancer statistic, where the literature might say that only one out a thousand patients experience negative symptoms from a particular drug?

What happens if you are that one statistic who suffers serious side effects? Most of my oncology doctors, even the better communicators, chose to ignore these discussions and downplay the side effects of the drugs prescribed, until I learned to insist on thorough information and disclosures.

My first oncologist won the prize for being the poorest and most negative communicator. She put me down repeatedly for what she called "oversensitivity" to drugs, as if I had control over my bad reactions to a long list of aromatase inhibitors and other drugs prescribed for my specific type of breast cancer.

In an email to me, she wrote, *"You have to take the drugs I prescribed. Live with the side effects; you have no choice. It's for your own good."* Without discussion, or any hint of concern, care, or humanity towards me, let alone living up to her physician's obligation to listen carefully to every patient, she repeatedly dismissed and ignored my reports on the extreme joint, muscle pain, stiffness, migraine headaches, stomach pains, and sleepless nights that I was experiencing from the cancer meds.

At times, I could hardly walk because of the pain and stiffness I was experiencing. I will never forget her unbelievable response when she very defensively told me, *"In all my (her) 15 years of practice, I never had a patient who reported any side effects from any of these drugs."* I found that hard to believe. Without further conversation, or attempt to explore other options with me, she tried to shut me up and let me know she was the expert-in-charge, and knew my body's tolerance level, better than I did. Her supercilious behavior was unacceptable.

It was another one of those mounting and reaffirming moments when I realized I had to take control. I knew my body's reactions better than any doctor. I had to step up and be my own best advocate. I responded to the doctor's email the next day and wrote:

"Dear Doctor, did you read the fine print in the literature provided by the pharmaceutical company, outlining the potentially negative and serious reactions from these drugs? These side effects I am experiencing are not in my head. They are real and getting worse. Every one of them is listed in the information packaged with the drug. Unfortunately, Doctor, I have been experiencing many of them for a long time, and you seem to be ignoring me."

Again, she responded very defensively and indifferently with an email filled with corporate-like jargon stating, *"Statistically, those are rare cases. I am a scientist, first and foremost, and I know what's good for you!"*

My nagging fear was confirmed. She was looking at me as just another cancer statistic. At that point, I desperately wanted to look her in the eyes, talk to her frankly, and make her understand I am not a statistic, rather a real person with unique reactions to certain drugs. I was forced instead to write her again since the 2020 COVID protocol she was strictly enforcing, prohibited me, even as her new cancer patient, from in-person meetings. I replied again asking her if she read the plethora of articles and literature from the pharmaceutical companies, clinical trials, and independent research reports that clearly cautioned patients, and I quoted, *"Immediately and openly discuss any side effects from the drug with your oncologist since side effects can be dangerous."*

Holy Moly, she did not acknowledge any of my concerns. She had a protective shield around her as impenetrable as the Federal Reserve Bank vault. She was a textbook case study on how a doctor should never respond. To make matters worse, she didn't stop there, but exasperated the matter, made my blood pressure rise, and followed up, yet again, with a very long email that said, in part summary, *"You are responsible for your own cancer. You wouldn't be in this situation if you had taken better care of yourself. You have to take these drugs, or I can't help you any longer."* Her language, not only sounded legally defensive, but was extremely offensive, and devoid of any understanding of what I was going through as her patient. She was also outrageously and unacceptably laying blame for cancer totally on me, adding a lot of stress to an already serious health crisis. At that moment, I decided to end my patient-doctor relationship with her.

It is often said that in darkness and pain there can be a silver lining. In my case, it was the much overdue big kick in the side of the pants, once again, to find another doctor with a more temperate ego, better listening skills, and patient-caring skills.

Like too many physicians, who are under strict institutional administrative time restraints, or maybe just overworked and burned-out, this physician in denial ignored the necessity of thoroughly understanding her patient's medical history and personal profile. She certainly didn't understand, or bother to learn how conscientious and proactive I had been all my life when it came to my healthcare and physical exercise. Her years of cancer practice hardened her to the point of extreme callousness and indifference—a medical malady contracted by many doctors, nurses and practitioners I encountered during my cancer journey.

I believe the only cure for this type of disease many physicians possess must involve examining and changing institutional practices and priorities that fail to put the patient first. Simply put, medical training hasn't caught up with the new and constantly evolving scientific knowledge about the mind-body connection. Mandatory training and the re-learning for every physician and medical practitioner has to take place. There can no longer be excuses for them to deny the importance of this critical connection in patient care, communications, and healing.

There is an old Indian proverb that says, "Never judge any man (woman) until you have walked two moons in his (her) moccasins." Every medical school and institution, not following and enforcing this scientifically verifiable body of medical research must be identified and called out. If it means rethinking and recalculating profitability, patient-doctor caseloads, changing time management rules, and the allowable amount of time a doctor can spend with her patients, it must be done. These institutions are failing you as a patient if they are not doing so.

A few doctors I met along the way, acknowledged the importance of my serious concerns about some of the major failings of traditional medicine. One culpable doctor frankly told me, "I have over 2,500 patients, and I just don't have the bandwidth to be as thorough as I would like to be." He told me this after he misdiagnosed my cancer for over a year and said it was frozen shoulder.

Hard-Learned Lesson:

Never second guess what your body is telling you. Never tolerate a doctor who doesn't treat you as a whole person, body, mind and spirit, and who doesn't listen to you carefully.

Check your own doctor's caseload at the beginning of your patient-doctor relationship.

Be ready to get another doctor at any point in your medical treatment if you are not getting the thorough care and professional treatment you deserve. There are definitely dedicated and caring doctors out there, but you have to do your homework and seek them out. Never be afraid to take appropriate action and report it.

6

HUMORLESS PRACTITIONERS & LAUGHTER THERAPY

"I'm so used to getting scans that the next time I go through airport security, I'm afraid I'll automatically lie down next to my bags going through screening."

—Mom

Cancer is no laughing matter, but you must try to find the joy in everyday living and keep smiling, whenever you can. Both medical literature and the Bible in

Proverbs 17:22 KJV agree, "A merry heart doeth good like a medicine, but a broken spirit doeth break the bones." According to the Mayo Clinic, one of the top medical centers, laughter can be a very effective remedy for healing.

Did you know a hardy laugh actually enhances your intake of oxygen-rich air, stimulates the heart, lungs and muscles, and helps the brain release endorphins, the body's natural painkillers? The best part is that good humor is free with no health insurance needed, can be self-administered, doesn't involve any uncomfortable injections, infusions, or claustrophobic imaging machines, and has no dangerous side effects. Even under the care of some sour and humorless practitioners, a big smile can raise your spirits and create a more positive healing environment, enabling you to face the ongoing drudgery and pain of cancer treatments.

During my medical battle, I discovered that friendly, joyful doctors and practitioners were a rarity. Rather, the didactic, uncaring and, sometimes, abrupt personalities of the staff were more common. Case in point, I was referred to a rheumatologist because of the extreme joint pain I was experiencing as a side effect of some of my medicines. When I entered the examining room, I greeted the doctor with a smile and a cheery "hello," and "how are you?" It was not reciprocated. Instead, he grumbled, "This is not a social visit. What are you here for?" I couldn't help but think this doctor didn't bother to read my medical chart and was probably trained by a disciple of Nurse Ratched, the cold, heartless, tyrannical fictional character, who became the stereotype for uncaring patient treatment in the psychological drama, "One Flew over the Cuckoo's Nest."

Despite this unfortunate reality which exists throughout today's healthcare institutions, a plethora of medical research and articles clearly indicate that good humor, joyful interactions and laughter are critical components in treating patients, particularly those battling cancer and serious diseases. The widespread acceptance and popular dissemination of this knowledge seem to have ended up in trash cans, or fallen on deaf ears.

I actually discovered that as early as the 1300s, Professor Henri de Mondeville successfully practiced laughter therapy with his patients with remarkable results. Norman Cousins, a well-known author and professor, in the 1980s developed his own laughter treatments in healing patients. In fact, applying his teachings to himself, he attributed his cure from a rare joint disease to continual laughter therapy treatments and fun activities. Astonishingly, he concluded that ten minutes of laughter, in ongoing intervals throughout the day, allowed him to be pain-free for two hours at a time. He kept teaching and laughing.

My own belief in the power of laughter has been strongly and continually reinforced by my brilliant, humorous and creative brother, Bob Basso. He is one of the most passionate advocates, authors and teachers of Laughter Therapy. He wrote several books on the positive impact of fun and laughter, and created a series of educational workshops on the subject. For years, he lectured at the University of California, Los Angeles (UCLA) as an instructor, and became a much in-demand speaker at hospitals and medical institutions throughout the United States. Featured on the front cover of People magazine, he was deservedly called, "America's Number One Fun Motivators." When applied in a medical setting, his teachings helped increase productivity, patient satisfaction, and decrease staff burn-out. More importantly, brother Bob has been one of the best friends, personal motivators and supporters God could have given to me. To this day, he brings constant color, light, joy, and laughter to my life.

Continuing to the present, the importance of laughter in healing has been backed up with ongoing scientific studies which prove laughter assists in the recovery process in treating cancer and other diseases by releasing the body's natural cancer-killing cells and shoring up the body's immune system. A recent study, conducted by the Washington University School of

Medicine in 2023, further highlights these important medical findings.

In the area of brain research, there have been a multitude of studies that underscore the fact that negative thoughts manifest into actual negative chemical reactions in the brain, which negatively affect the body by creating stress and decreasing immunity. In contrast, these reports show that positive and happy thoughts release neuropeptides, the body's natural healers, and help fight stress and serious illnesses.

I also recently discovered that an increasing number of top medical hospitals, like the University of California, San Francisco (UCSF) now offer courses in Laughter Therapy and healing. In India, Laughter Yoga has also been a long-time healing remedy used with great success.

Unfortunately, communicating and applying this cogent information on the critical importance of the healing power of laughter, hasn't been a priority in medical facilities in the United States, nor seriously taught in the training of physicians and technicians. It seems officious and humorless doctors, practitioners and clinicians still hold onto the obsolete idea that fun and laughter in a medical environment diminishes their importance, reputation and efficacy in patient treatment, which is definitely far from the truth. Doctors should comfortably embrace the fact that it is a critical part of medical treatment and, at minimum, creates a healthy healing environment.

I get it! Doctors are focused on a gazillion diseases, and trained to deal with endless medical maladies and symptoms, but never should they forget that they are dealing with a whole human being, complete with body, mind and spirit, not just a disease.

So where does that leave cancer warriors who don't have a special brother, or teacher who can nourish them with the power of joy and laughter? You must find support and more *functional* medical centers that fully understand and apply these principles based on holistic medicine. Go online to visit the website for The Institute for Functional Medicine (*www.ifm.org*), and in the search bar, google "find a functional medical doctor in my (your) area". The best test to determine if your doctors and practitioners are treating you as a whole person, with full knowledge of your unique individual needs, is your actual encounters with your doctor, and pay attention to your gut feelings. In your early interactions and treatment with your doctors, if it doesn't feel right; it is probably not right!

Hard-Learned Lesson:

Don't ever let yourself be taken down by negative practitioners and equally dire medical environments. Never succumb to negative thinking, or the joyless communications of any doctor, or healthcare worker. Remind them in a respectful but assertive manner, you're ultimately in control of your health and healing.

Seek out fun, joyful and happy friends, experiences and activities. Gather an army of positive and cheerful supporters. Immediately, erase all negative thinking and eliminate negative people from your life. When you slip into destructive thinking, stop yourself by repeating the phrase, "I am positive, I am happy, and I will do everything possible to stay in control of my thoughts, actions and healing."

7

TRUE LOVE & FURRY FRIENDS

"The world would be a nicer place if everyone learned to love as unconditionally as a dog."

—M.K. Clinton

It took cancer and thirty plus years of marriage to fully realize my husband, Charles, is my real knight in shining armor. He earned the title, not based on his good looks, soft penetrating crystal blue eyes, constant upbeat spirit, crazy sense of humor, incredible work ethic, talent and sense of responsibility, but because he stands by my side day and night, doctor visit after visit, medical test after test, emergency after emergency, during thick and thin. Our wedding vows, "In sickness and health, for better or worse, until death do we part," meant something to him. He proves it over and over again every day.

With over fifty percent of marriages ending in divorce, often occurring during trouble times, I am blessed. I told Charles if things get worse for me, I don't want to be a burden to him, so he can divorce me now while I am still standing. He replied, "Not on your life!" So, we moved on facing the herculean cancer challenge, head-on! We now have a standing joke. When it's time for Charles to drive me to another doctor's appointment, he says, "Driving Miss Daisy, today!" We always laugh, and I think of the great patience and aplomb, the iconic actor, Morgan Freeman, portrayed in "Driving Miss Daisy," as the chauffeur in that memorable movie. Driving me hither and yonder, Charles' unflappable spirit and humor always keeps the mood light, making my doctor visits almost pleasant!

When we met it was definitely "like" at first sight. There was something about his energy that drew me to him. We were two strangers that met at the Los Angeles Airport, simply waiting for a shuttle bus. Charles had a big white bandage on his head due to a minor surgery, so I couldn't really see his whole face. He just arrived in LA to train an actor in martial arts. Dressed in my most colorful sarong, I was just off a flight from a vacation in the Hawaiian island of Molokai. We were the most unlikely soon-to-be couple. His striking crystal-blue eyes were the only thing I saw, but it was his genuine big smile and happy demeanor that ignited our first conversation. Shortly, the shuttle bus arrived and, not coincidentally, we sat next to each other. Now, thirty plus years after, the mutual "like" we first experienced, turned into genuine love.

It is amazing how freely the word "love" is bantered around with the young, the married, the old, and the Hollywood crowd, but I believe it takes a real life challenge, or struggle, such as a life-and-death situation, to understand and achieve real love. We were both unfortunate that cancer invaded our home, but, at the same time, blessed to be able to meet the challenge and continue to grow in love.

On April 8, 2020, as if it were yesterday, I remember standing in the hallway of our house, greeting Charles coming home from work.

He said, "What's up, you like you were crying?" I blurted out the news that the doctor just confirmed I had metastatic breast cancer. We stood in the hallway crying and tightly embracing each other. It seemed like hours had passed; we were still crying like babies, in between Charles' reassuring hugs and comments, telling me, "Don't worry, I'm here for you always, and you will not fight this battle alone. You will win. We will win, together!"

With Charles' help and continual encouragement, in addition to following the prescribed standard treatment of my new more humane oncologist,

I kept an open mind, researched, and explored alternative approaches to curing cancer. Then, out of the blue one day, I received a call from a dear old high school friend who tracked me down from New York, where we grew up. Impeccable timing! What a coincidence! It just so happened that her husband studied and practiced Chinese medicine. When I told her about my current health condition, she strongly advised that I visit with a holistic practitioner she knew in Marin County in California. On the reference of my trusted friend, with great hope and a little curiosity, I made an appointment.

What was totally remarkable about my appointment with this herbalist was not just the ton of herbs and vitamins he prescribed, written in unreadable Chinese characters, but the mysterious encounter I had with his dog.

As I entered his waiting room, checked in at the front desk, and sat down, a beautiful golden Labrador retriever stood up from his resting position, stared at me intensely, and slowly started walking toward me.

When he reached my side, without looking for pats on his head, or any acknowledgement whatsoever, he sat a few feet beside me, and didn't move until the doctor came out to get me.

When I followed the doctor into his office, the dog very closely trailed me and laid beside me. Quite puzzled, I asked the doctor why his dog was following me. He said, "Did you recently receive an unpleasant medical diagnosis?" I told him my doctor told me a few weeks ago that I had breast cancer. Letting out a big sigh, he commented, "I am glad you already know."

Charles and I were stunned. The doctor proceeded to tell us that his dog, Brandy, was among an elite group of canines who were carefully selected to receive special training to identify and sniff out cancer and other diseases, and with his extensive training, he is almost hundred percent accurate in his assessments. I remained speechless for a few more minutes, amazed at the incredible ability of our furry friends. These magnificent animals, with proper training, whether on the battlefield, or in police work, or in an alternative holistic medical facility, can identify danger and many diseases.

I took many of the herbs the doctor prescribed and continued my immunotherapy with my traditional oncologist. To this day, I remain in awe of Brandy's keen olfactory senses.

When we arrived home that day, as always, we were more than gleefully greeted by my two most loving and overly rambunctious dogs, Daisy, a Maltese, and Bella, a Poodle mix. I gave them the biggest hugs. At that instance, Charles looked at me and said, "Do you think that's why Bella stays at your side all the time, day and night, even when you go to the shower, dress, eat, sleep, or whatever? She is glued to you!" Even though Bella was certainly not trained, and resists directions of any kind, I couldn't help but think that as a member of a special canine class of God's creatures, bestowed with a superior sense of smell, Bella may very well sense cancer in my body. Since then, I read numerous well-documented articles about how some dogs possess the ability to warn their owners about pending diabetic shock and other medical emergencies. Unquestionably, I have a heightened sense of gratitude and love for all our furry friends.

Hard-Learned Lesson:

Live a life of gratitude.

Hug your husband and loved ones often, and continually thank them for all the things they do for you, both on and off the "honey-do-list."

Dogs are God's precious gifts to us, furnishing us with endless affection, devotion, and constantly teaching us what unconditional love and loyalty really are. Indeed, they seem to have all the virtues and none of the vices of the human species.

8
PRAY, PRAY & PRAY MORE

"For truly I tell you, if you have faith the size of a mustard seed, you will say to this mountain, 'Move from here to there,' and it will move; nothing will be impossible for you."

—Matthew 17:20-21

Why do we turn to God when we are in need? For many of us, it is a subconscious admission that there is someone more powerful than ourselves. For cancer warriors, I believe it has to be a conscious and deliberate acknowledgment you can't fight cancer, the biggest monster of your lifetime, alone.

I prayed a lot as a child and continued into adulthood, but, admittedly, not with as much mindfulness, or frequency as when I was under the tutelage of the good nuns back at St. Pancras Grammar School. Thinking back to childhood, praying was really a conditioned response, part of my Catholic upbringing and training. To prove my point, a bizarre thing happened one Sunday after Church when my family went to see the then popular movie, "Ole Yeller." As I entered the theatre row to go to my seat, I automatically genuflected and performed the traditional sign of the cross on my forehead and chest, thinking I was entering the Church pew. My Mom tripped over me in the dark theatre, the popcorn she was carrying went flying all over, and the rest of the family laughed uncontrollably, disturbing the entire movie house. To this day at family gatherings, this embarrassing childhood story somehow seems to warrant a retelling, and never fails to get a burst of laughter.

Every year in grammar school when it was my assigned turn for family prayer time, I brought home the over-sized school rosary that barely fit into my school bag. On a continual rotational schedule, each family in the parish had to take the rosary home for a week. The thought was that if the parishioners were in constant prayer, blessings and good things would happen to them. As a kid, I believed community prayer would create beneficial effects, but, readily admit, it never stopped some awful things from happening. It didn't prevent the rowdy boys from tearing up the school playground and harassing the girls, never stopped the neighborhood Rottweiler from terrorizing the Good Humor ice cream man every time he heard the distinct bell, nor did it fend off the annual snowstorms, hurricanes and flu.

When it was my family's turn to bring home the rosary, we would gather in the living room, turn off the nightly news on our RCA TV console, and one by one, wooden bead by wooden bead, make our way around the beads and pray.

We recited five sets of Hail Mary's on the smaller beads and five Our Father's on the larger ones since we were instructed to say the entire rosary every night for seven days. Dutifully, the family did so every night the prayer beads were in our possession. Sometimes my Dad, who was a fireman at the time, would excuse himself because he would come home from work, covered with smoke, soot and all kinds of debris, totally exhausted from putting out 5-alarm fires in New York City's towering infernos. Later on when he rose to the top of his rank and became a Chief in the New York City Fire Department, I believed our prayers helped, but, without question, it was his indefatigable nightly studying and endless pounding away at his books that eventually got him to top spot. Dad always said, "Prayer is important, but first you have to do the hard work to achieve your goals." He proved it by the way he lived.

In those days, I really thought of God as a miracle worker, a sort of Santa Claus who generously bestowed good things, provided us with the things we wanted, and forgave our sins, on demand. Particularly around Christmas time, I remember innocently, but selfishly, praying, "Dear Lord, I was a good girl this year so please give me the things I am praying for?" Then, item by item, I would shamelessly list all my must-haves from clothes to games to whatever was the talking, walking trendy item of the season.

It wasn't until decades later when I got cancer that I realized the importance, true power, comfort, and spiritual connection to God that deep intentional prayer provided. I no longer prayed for material possessions, but for the strength, guidance and courage to fight the "big C." To this day, with absolute fervor, I pray continually when I'm in pain, when I can't sleep, when I'm stuck in a PET scan and MRI, or when I am anxiously waiting for the results from my regular three-month medical check-up to see if the cancer has further metastasized.

It's an incredible feeling of lightness, just being in the present, talking to a higher power. I become relaxed, and, more importantly, closer to God, knowing, without any doubt, that God is the most caring, understanding friend and companion anyone could wish for on a challenging journey.

While I believe God can perform miracles, I also realize that alone we have little control to change anything, let along stop the potential progression of those insidious cancer cells, eating away at the various parts of our bodies. I voraciously read spiritual books to make sure I continually get all the reinforcement I need to maintain a positively healthy mindset.

A life-long friend, Michael Anthony, who embraced a spiritual path in life, wrote a book on the keys to mental strength, and furnished me with dozens more on faith, prayer and miracles. These immensely inspirational books provided me with the psychological and spiritual ammunition needed to deal with daily health challenges. Michael's own book: "How To Be Happy and Have Fun Changing the World," is a powerful testament that all positive change must begin with one's self. To have a healthy and happy life, he builds a compelling case in his book that it is imperative to have positive thoughts and eliminate all negative thinking, no matter what monsters come your way.

In today's topsy-turvy world, when most everyone is faced with some kind of health or life challenge, I often think Michael's book is a must-read. His words of advice are a powerful reminder that if you change your thinking, attitude and actions, you can positively help change a negative situation, begin to see problems in a different light, and potentially even experience better mental and physical health.

As a powerful daily spiritual reminder, I carry in my wallet the inspiring allegorical poem, "Footprints in the Sand" which reads:

One night I dreamed I was walking

along the beach with the Lord. Many scenes

from my life flashed across the sky.

In each scene I noticed footprints in the sand. Sometimes there were two footprints, other times there were only one.

This bothered me because I noticed during the low periods of my life when I was suffering from anxiety, sorrow or defeat, I could see only one set of footprints, so I said to the Lord,

"You promised me Lord that if I followed you, you would walk with me always. But I have noticed during the most trying periods of my life there has been only one set of footprints in the sand. Why when I needed you most, have you not been there for me?"

The Lord replied, "The years that you have seen only one set of footprints, my child, is when I carried you."

These reassuring words are priceless gems which help ignite the spark in my daily life, give me the strong incentive to get up in the morning, and provide a healthy dose of spiritual medicine for my soul.

I even programmed my Android phone to a prayer app which reminds me by way of a gentle buzz throughout the day to stop whatever I am doing and pray. When I first set my mobile phone up, I had a big chuckle, along with the friends I told about my new-found app because hands-down, I am among the least tech-savvy twenty-first century humans whose birth pre-dated the age of computers, the internet and apps.

It is amazing how this one prayer app far outweighs all the misinformation and trash on the internet!

Hard-Learned Lesson:

Cancer cannot silence your prayers. Without question, the biggest lesson of my ongoing cancer journey is that God is your best ally.

Pray. Pray often. Pray deeply. Miracles do happen. But, remember, as you traverse the many labyrinths of the healthcare system, first, you have to do the hard work of becoming your own best advocate. If you are not able to do so, make sure you have a good friend or family member who can help you.

After four years since my metastatic breast cancer diagnosis, I am still very blessed, living on Earth, and enjoying simple pleasures. Occasionally, I can even be heard humming a verse from an old song, "Cruising down the river on a Sunday afternoon," a happy tune my Mom taught me when I was a very young child.

AFTERWORD

Bring "My Little Pink Notebook: How To Be Your Own Best Advocate Fighting Cancer & Other Monsters," which I wrote especially for you, to all your doctor appointments. Take very good notes in the pages provided at the back of this book. My sincere hope and prayer is that you may benefit in some way from my experiences and insights.

Stay Positive! Stay Strong! God Bless!

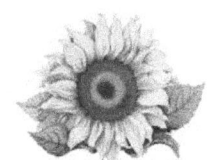

NOTES

www.ingramcontent.com/pod-product-compliance
Lightning Source LLC
LaVergne TN
LVHW011727060526
838200LV00051B/3057